The Body-Mind-World Connection

Rethinking Illness and Wellness

Freudian Trips

Copyright Page

Disclaimer

The views and opinions expressed in this book are those of
the author(s) and do not necessarily reflect the official policy
or position of any other agency, organization, employer, or
company. The contents of this book are for informational and
educational purposes only and are not intended to serve as
professional advice, diagnosis, or treatment.

The information provided in this book is believed to be
accurate and reliable as of the date of publication. However, it
may include some errors or inaccuracies, and no warranty or
guarantee is provided regarding the accuracy, timeliness, or
applicability of the content.

Readers are encouraged to consult with professional
philosophers, educators, or other qualified professionals
where appropriate for personalized advice. The author(s) and
publisher shall not be liable for any loss, damage, or harm
caused or alleged to be caused, directly or indirectly, by the

information or ideas contained, suggested, or referenced in this book.

By reading this book, the reader acknowledges and agrees that they are solely responsible for how they interpret and apply the information contained herein.

This book may also include references to other works, studies, and sources. These references are provided for further reading and exploration and do not imply endorsement or validation of the specific theories, viewpoints, or interpretations presented in those works.

Introduction: A New Way to Understand Health

For a long time, doctors and scientists looked at the body like a machine. If something broke – a bone, an organ, even a tiny chemical process inside a cell – that was the cause of all your problems. This way of thinking is called the "biomedical model," and while it's been incredibly helpful for treating many diseases, it has its limits.

Imagine your car just won't start one day. The biomedical model is like taking it to the mechanic and only focusing on the engine. Sure, a faulty part might be the issue, but what if you're out of gas? Or the battery's dead? All those other factors matter, but they're easy to miss if you're only looking under the hood.

That's where Dr. George Engel stepped in. He realized that our health is just like that unreliable car. Our bodies are amazing but complicated machines. However, we're more than just biology. Our thoughts, feelings, and the world around us – these play a huge role in whether we're healthy or not. He called this wider, more complete picture the "Biopsychosocial Model."

The Biopsychosocial Model says we can't fix the car by only looking at the engine. We need to consider the whole picture:

- **Biological:** The actual workings of our bodies – genes, cells, organs.
- **Psychological:** Our minds – thought patterns, emotions, how we handle stress.
- **Social:** The environment – family, friends, jobs, where we live, how much money we have.

All these pieces can make us well or unwell. This approach offers a deeper understanding of why we get sick and leads to treatments that work better because they don't just target the faulty engine part, they consider the whole person.

Chapter 1: Our Body's Story – The Building Blocks of Health

Imagine your body is a magnificent house. This house is built from tiny blueprints called genes, passed down from your parents. These blueprints make you unique – the color of your eyes, your height, even how easily you get sunburned! But sometimes, these blueprints have tiny errors that make your house more prone to problems – maybe the roof is a little leaky, making you more likely to get colds. That's the idea of genetics and how it affects our health.

Your house also has special systems for keeping you safe and healthy:

- **The Command Center (The Nervous System):** Think of this as your house's electrical wiring, with your brain as the main control panel. It sends messages throughout your body, telling your heart to beat, your lungs to breathe, and keeping everything in check.

- **The Defense System (The Immune System):** This is like your house's security team. It fights off intruders like germs and viruses trying to cause trouble. Sometimes, this system gets overprotective and starts attacking things that aren't harmful, leading to allergies or other problems.
- **The Chemical Messengers (Hormones and More):** These are like tiny mail carriers running around your house. Hormones are powerful chemicals that travel through your blood, affecting how you feel, grow, and even how much energy you have. If these messengers get mixed up, it can throw your whole house out of whack!

Sometimes, things inside your house aren't perfectly balanced. Maybe a pipe bursts (injury), or the power goes out (illness). Understanding how these systems work and how they sometimes go wrong is the first step in learning how to keep our 'body house' in tip-top shape.

Chapter 2: Mind Matters – Your Thoughts as Medicine (or Trouble!)

Imagine your thoughts are like the weather inside your 'body house' from the last chapter. Some days it's sunny and bright, other times it can be stormy and dark. Turns out, this inner weather has a huge impact on your health!

- **The Stress Storm:** When you're worried, scared, or overwhelmed, it sets off alarms in your brain. This is great for escaping real danger, but when it happens too often, it's like a constant storm battering your house. Headaches, stomachaches, and trouble sleeping are all signs that the stress storm is doing damage.
- **Feelings that Heal (or Hurt):** Emotions aren't just in your head. Sadness can make you feel tired and achy, anger can make your heart race, and happiness can feel like a warm glow. Sometimes, the bad feelings get so strong and the storms so frequent that they can lead to things like depression or anxiety.

- **The Power of Belief:** Have you ever felt sick just because you were worried about getting sick? Or gotten better simply because you believed a medicine would work? Our minds are powerful! What we think and expect can actually change how our bodies feel.

Think about it like this: if your 'house' constantly expects a burglar, you'll always be tense and on edge, even if no one is trying to break in! Learning how to calm your mind, handle strong feelings, and change negative thought patterns is like building stronger walls and a better alarm system – it keeps you safer and your 'body house' in better shape.

Chapter 3: Beyond the Body: How the World Shapes Our Health

Remember that incredible 'body house' we've been talking about? Well, it doesn't exist in a vacuum. Where that house is built, who lives nearby, and the kind of neighborhood it's in all have a huge impact on its condition.

- **Money Matters:** Imagine two houses. One has easy access to fresh food, a nearby gym, and a safe space for kids to play. The other is in a neighborhood with few healthy options and dangers on the streets. It's clear which house is going to be healthier, right? Unfortunately, not everyone has the same resources, and that impacts everything from heart disease to how long you live.
- **The Family Tree of Health:** Our family and culture teach us what 'normal' is. If everyone around you smokes, eats unhealthy foods, and avoids doctors, chances are you'll do the same. Changing these patterns can be hard, but it can lead to better health for you and future generations!

- **A Hug or a Hit:** Imagine two kids who get into a bike accident. One has parents who rush them to the hospital, offer comfort, and make sure they heal. The other gets yelled at, and maybe their wound isn't properly cared for. Both kids have physical injuries, but the emotional support (or lack of it) also impacts how quickly and fully they recover. And this pattern of love and support, or stress and hardship, lasts a lifetime.
- **When Bad Things Happen:** Big events like accidents, abuse, or living through a war can leave invisible scars. These affect our bodies and minds long after the original danger is gone. It's like your house was in an earthquake – even when the shaking stops, the damage remains. Getting the right kind of help can lead to healing, even years later.

The world around us isn't something that happens *to* us; it's part of our overall health picture. Making healthy places to live, supporting families, and creating safe, caring communities is like building a better neighborhood for everyone's 'body house'.

Chapter 4: Healing Stories – Putting the Puzzle Together

Imagine your health is a giant puzzle. The traditional approach to medicine focuses on just one or two pieces – the broken bone, the faulty heart valve. The Biopsychosocial Model helps doctors and patients see the whole picture. Here's how it changes lives:

- **The Pain Puzzle:** Sarah has been struggling with back pain for years. Doctors found some disc problems, but even after surgery, she still hurts. Her new team looks broader: her sleep is terrible, she's stressed by a difficult job, and memories of an old car accident make her tense up. Treatment now involves fixing her sleep routine, stress management techniques, and special therapy to release those old fears – alongside the physical care for her back.
- **The Heart's Worries:** Mr. Jones had a heart attack. He takes his medications faithfully, but he's still exhausted and scared it will happen again. A Biopsychosocial approach reveals he's depressed,

isolated since retiring, and convinced that being sick means he's helpless. Alongside heart rehab, he gets counseling, joins a senior center, and works on changing those negative thought patterns. His heart gets stronger, but also his spirit.

- **Feeling Better Inside and Out:** Lisa has struggled with anxiety since she was a kid. It causes stomachaches, headaches, and trouble focusing. Instead of just medication, she learns breathing exercises to calm down, how to face scary situations gradually, and explores the stressful patterns in her family that make things worse. Slowly, her body symptoms lessen as her mind learns new skills.
- **Breaking Free from Addiction:** Addiction isn't just about a substance – it changes your brain chemistry, but also fills a hole created by pain, trauma, or lack of connection. True recovery, using the Biopsychosocial Model, means detox and medications when needed, but also therapy to heal old wounds, developing life skills, and finding healthier community and support.

The Biopsychosocial Model doesn't mean ignoring medical problems. It means seeing that broken leg, faulty heart, troubled mind, or addictive craving as part of a greater whole. Just like solving a puzzle takes putting all the pieces together, it gives us the best chance for true, lasting healing.

Chapter 5: You're the Expert: Healing as a Partnership

Imagine going to a mechanic who never listens when you describe the strange sounds your car makes, fixes only one thing, and then sends you on your way. Frustrating, right? Unfortunately, that's how medicine sometimes works! The Biopsychosocial Model aims to change that.

- **You Know Your 'House' Best:** Imagine taking the mechanic on a ride, pointing out the squeaks, rattles, and places where it's struggling. That's what happens when doctors and other healthcare providers truly listen. You're the expert on your own body, how your mind works, and what your life's challenges are. This approach values your input and puts you at the center of your own care.
- **A Blueprint for Success:** When you and your medical team see the whole health picture, treatment plans make more sense! Maybe it's not *just* medication for your headaches, but also addressing your sleep troubles and tense work environment. When you're

part of the planning process, you're more likely to stick with treatments that truly target all the causes, not just the symptoms.

- **Body, Mind, and Spirit Matter:** Sometimes people feel shame when they're told, "It's all in your head," as if their problems aren't real. The Biopsychosocial Model says, "Your head *is* real!" Mental health is just as important as physical health. When it's okay to talk about depression, stress, or past trauma as part of your care, everyone can address issues that might be stopping you from fully healing.

Think of it like this: your 'body house' needs a team of experts. Doctors and specialists know the structural stuff, but you're the resident who's lived there the longest. When everyone collaborates – the plumber, the electrician, the interior designer, and you at the center – the result is a home that's not just fixed, but the most comfortable and healthy it can be.

Chapter 6: Building a Better System – The Future of Healing

Imagine if every 'body house' had a full, expert team assigned – not just the plumber (the surgeon) and electrician (the specialist), but experts on stress, the mind, lifestyle, and the neighborhood it's in. That's the potential of the Biopsychosocial Model! Here's what it might look like:

- **The Dream Team:** Maybe you're seeing a doctor for high blood pressure. Instead of just pills, your team could include a nutritionist to help with healthy eating, a therapist for stress management, or even a social worker if money problems are making it hard to get good food. This means attacking the problem from all sides!
- **Training Camp for Health Heroes:** Doctors, nurses, therapists, and everyone involved in health need training in all parts of the Biopsychosocial Model. That means understanding how poverty affects health, how the mind can help or harm the body, AND all the medical science they already know.

- **A Health Hub, Not Just a Hospital:** Imagine a clinic that's not just for sick visits. It could offer classes on managing stress, healthy cooking, support groups, and even have lawyers or financial specialists to help with those issues that impact health. This makes care about prevention as much as fixing what's already broken

Think of it like this: Right now, treating your whole health picture is like doing a complicated home improvement project yourself. You have to find all the specialists, coordinate everything, and hope they communicate. The Biopsychosocial Model is like hiring a trustworthy general contractor to make your healthy 'house' remodel a breeze.

It won't be an easy change. It requires rethinking how we pay for healthcare, train practitioners, and create new types of clinics. But the potential is amazing – a system designed to keep people truly well, not just patch them up when things go wrong.

Conclusion: A Health Revolution – It Starts with You

We've taken a journey together. You've seen how your 'body house' isn't just a bundle of bones and organs. Your mind, your experiences, the world around you – all of it shapes your wellbeing. The Biopsychosocial Model isn't just a fancy term, it's a powerful idea: Healing happens best when we address the whole person.

Imagine a world where:

- Doctors listen to your whole story, not just your symptoms.
- Mental health is considered as crucial as a healthy heart.
- Communities are designed to support health, not make us sick.

This isn't some far-off dream. It's happening, little by little. But it needs your voice! Here's how you can be part of the change:

- **Advocate for Yourself:** Ask questions about your care. Don't be afraid to mention the stress in your life or the sadness you feel alongside a physical problem. Demand that your medical team sees you as a whole person.
- **Seek Holistic Care:** Look for doctors, therapists, and clinics that embrace the philosophy of the Biopsychosocial Model. These practitioners will partner with you for better health.
- **Spread the Word:** Tell your friends, family, and community about this approach. The more people understand that the mind, body, and world are connected when it comes to health, the more they'll demand a healthcare system that reflects those values.

Remember, your 'body house' is the only one you'll ever have. The Biopsychosocial Model offers the tools to make it a place of strength, health, and resilience, from the inside out. Let's build a healthier future, together.

About Freudian Trips

Welcome to Freudian Trips, your dedicated platform for diving deep into the world of psychology. We are more than just a YouTube channel or a book publisher. We are a beacon of enlightenment, making complex psychological concepts accessible and engaging for all.

Our YouTube channel is a rich repository of psychology made simple. We take the profound and often complex ideas from the world of psychology and break them down into digestible, easy-to-understand content. From the foundational theories of Freud to the cognitive insights of Piaget, we cover a broad spectrum of psychological schools and thoughts, making psychology accessible to everyone, regardless of their background or prior knowledge.

As a book publisher, we take the same approach, transforming intricate psychological theories into comprehensible narratives. Our books are not just collections of words, but vessels of wisdom that make psychology approachable and relatable. We believe that psychology should not be confined to academic circles, but should be available to all who seek to understand the human mind and behavior.

At Freudian Trips, we believe in the power of curiosity and the pursuit of knowledge. We are here to stoke the fires of your curiosity, to guide you on your intellectual journey, and to help you navigate the fascinating world of psychology.

If you are someone who is not afraid to question, to explore, and to learn, then you are in the right place. Join us on this journey of exploration, as we make psychology easy to understand, one concept at a time.

Be sure to visit our Youtube channel at:
www.freudiantrips.com/youtube

You can also visit us on the web at www.freudiantrips.com

Welcome to The Freudian Trip community. Stay curious. Stay enlightened.